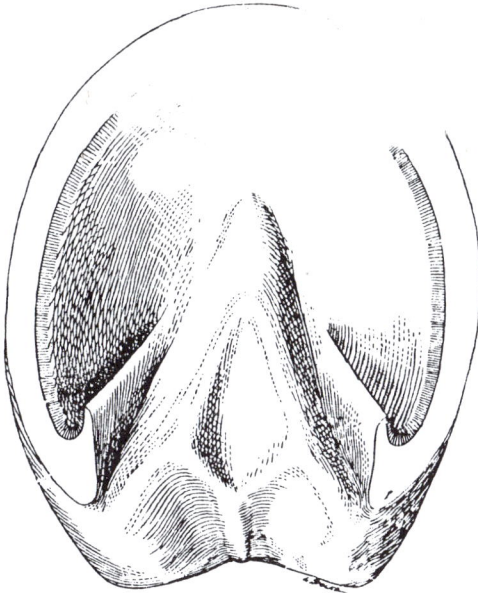

HORSE
FOOT
CARE

by Doug Butler, PhD, CJF, FWCF
Doug Butler Enterprises, Inc.
P.O. Box 1390
LaPorte, CO 80535
1-800-728-3826

ISBN number: 0-916992-15-2

Toe

Wall

Sole

White line

Point of frog

Quarter

Commissure

Seat of corn

Bar

Cleft of frog

Heel

Buttress of heel

Bulb

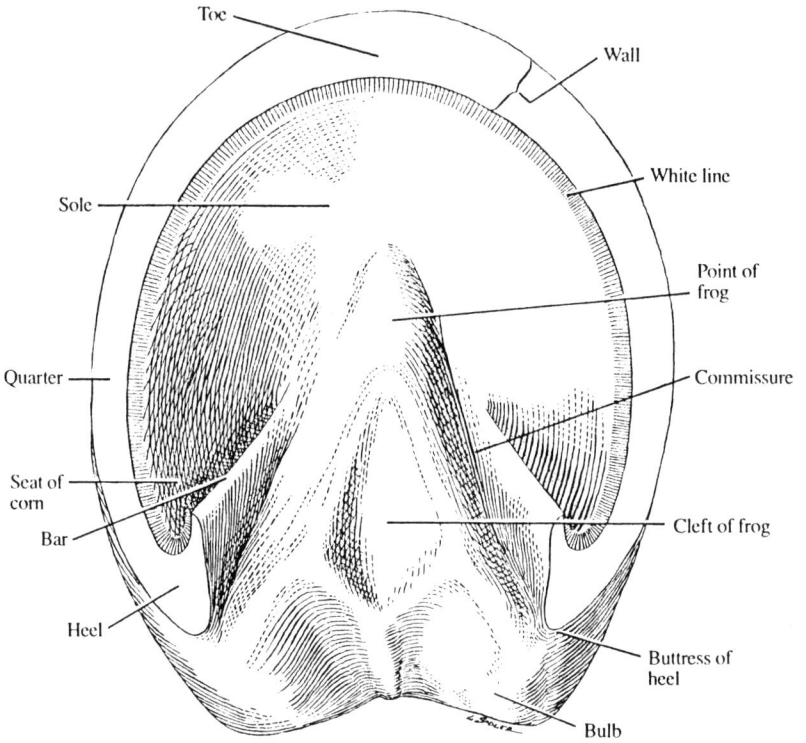

The parts of the hoof

INTRODUCTION

Modern domesticated horses depend entirely upon humans for their maintenance and health. Horses are living beings with feelings and are subject to many ailments that affect their well being and usefulness to their human partners.

The information in this book will help you provide humane foot care for your horse. This information, when used consistently, will help prevent needless suffering as well as inconvenience due to lameness caused by neglect, misunderstanding, or lack of knowledge.

Horse Foot Care will guide you in providing humane hoof care for your horse. You will learn the basic vocabulary needed to understand horses' feet and to discuss problems with horse care professionals—farriers and veterinarians.

Before purchasing a horse, have a competent farrier as well as an equine veterinarian examine the horse. Purchase it only if these experts pronounce it sound. This is especially true when you're considering buying an expensive performance athlete. Pet or infrequently ridden pleasure horses may tolerate foot problems that could prevent a competitive athlete from giving its best performance.

Horse ownership should be an enjoyable experience, but a lame horse can cast a dark cloud over what ought to be a beautiful experience. The foot is the horse's foundation, and foot problems cause the majority of lamenesses. Thus the ancient adage: no foot —no horse.

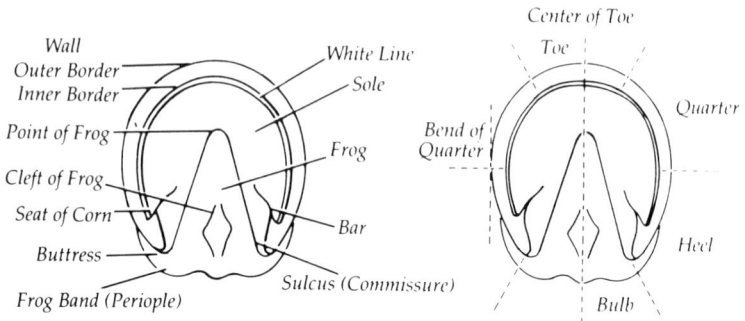

The parts of the hoof

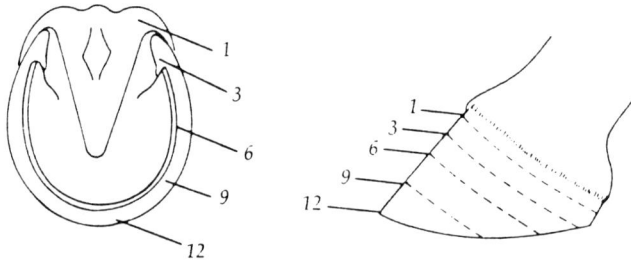

The growth and age of the hoof wall (in months)

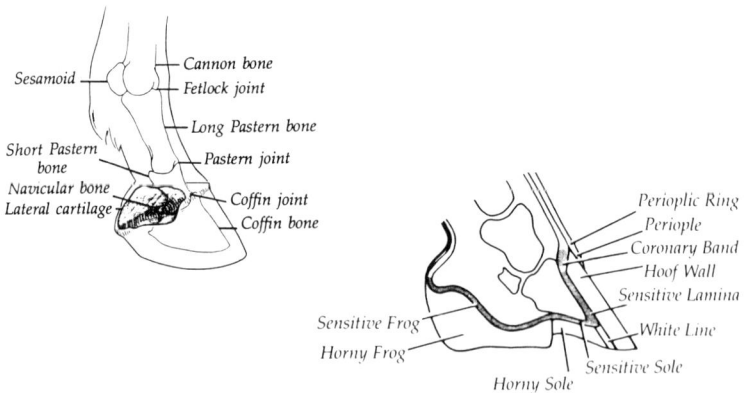

The relationship of sensitive structures to hoof structures

FOOT STRUCTURE AND FUNCTION

The foot of the horse is defined as the hoof and its contents. Each foot is uniquely designed to support weight, resist wear, replenish itself, absorb shock, provide traction, conduct moisture and assist in pumping venous blood. The foot must be healthy to operate at peak efficiency and must receive proper care to remain sound.

The hoof wall bears the weight of the horse (see pg 30). The lamina attaches the hoof wall to the coffin bone and transfers the horse's weight from the bone to the hoof.

The hoof wall grows downward from the coronary band. Hoof wall growth averages 3/8 inch per month, but is faster during the late spring season and when a horse is young.

The white line is a buffer between the movements of the sole and the wall. It is the guideline for hoof shaping and nail placement. The sole protects the internal structures of the foot from injury. The frog absorbs shock and provides traction. Movements of the foot assist in pumping blood back to the heart.

Hoof conformation has a great effect on a horse's predisposition to foot disease. Each time a horse is trimmed and shod, its foot must be balanced by the farrier so that the body weight will be evenly distributed over the foot.

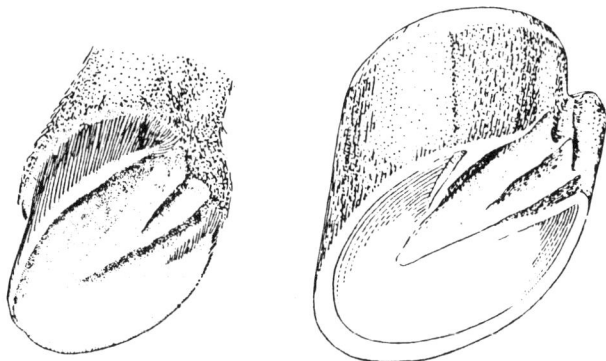

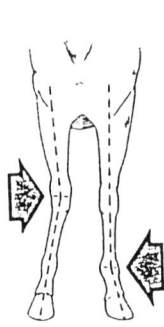 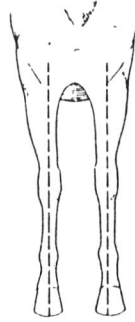

Neglected   *Cared For*

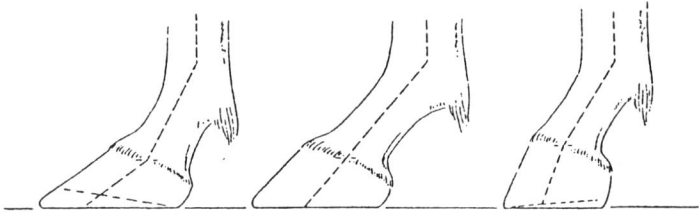

Broken Back   *Correct*   *Broken Forward*

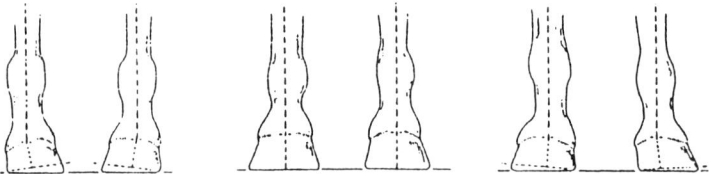

Broken Out   *Straight*   *Broken In*

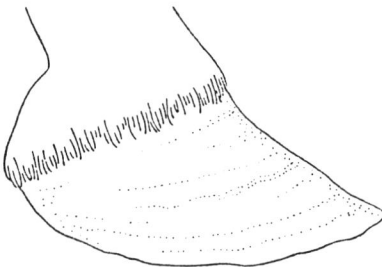 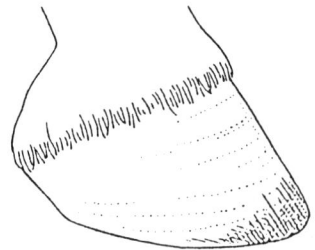

Before   *After*

HOOF MANAGEMENT

Good management is the best way to prevent foot problems.

Healthy, balanced hoofs maximize the many important functions of horse feet. Horses with ideal conformation and hoofs proportional to the horse's body size allow ideal distribution of body weight over the surface area of the hoof. A regularly balanced foot (shod or unshod) is an important part of good manangement. Hoofs should normally be trimmed or shod every 6 to 8 weeks.

More frequent hoof trimming (every 4 weeks) is especially important in young horses when the bones are growing. Handle foals regularly, training them from birth to accept eventual farrier work. Treat crooked limbs as early as possible with the farrier and veterinarian working together.

Make the environment for the horse as safe as possible. Keep loose barbed wire, machinery and other sharp objects away from horses. Failure to pay attention to the safety of the area where you keep your horses can result in serious wounds to the foot (and other parts of the body). Immunize your horses against tetanus every year to protect them from this disease which may develop from foot injury infections.

Feed containing all the nutrients a horse needs (such as good quality hay and salt) produces maximum hoof growth and quality. Use grain such as clean oats only to maintain weight, especially when doing hard work. Unless the horse's ration is of extremely poor quality or the horse lives in a nutrient deficient area, feeding the animal expensive feed supplements cannot be justified. It is usually more practical to buy higher quality feed ingredients.

Exercise helps to circulate blood containing essential nutrients to the hoof. The ground surface also affects the quality of the hoof. (Dry rocky ground normally strengthens horses' feet.)

The best place to keep your horses is a green pasture; if that isn't possible, a dry feed lot is the next best option. A stable is the least desirable unless it is kept clean, is well-ventilated, and the horse is worked daily. You can improve a dry lot by overflowing the water trough to create a muddy area around it.

Commercial hoof dressings have little or no beneficial effect on the hoofs of well-managed horses. Green pastures supply adequate Vitamin A necessary for hoof growth. You may need to provide Vitamin A supplement if you feed your horses brown hay over an extended time and you keep your horses in a stable.

Horses are creatures of habit and are sensitive to sudden changes in feed amounts or composition. Feed them at nearly the same time each day to prevent digestive upsets. Make changes in feeds over a period of several days. Reduce the grain portion of a working horse's ration by two-thirds on days the horse is idle to prevent colic or azoturia. Colic often produces laminitis or founder.

You can prevent many foot diseases by routine attention to hoof condition. Cleaning the feet out before and after riding is especially important. Watch for subtle changes in the horse's posture or gait; these will alert you to the need for closer examination. Regular visits by the farrier and veterinarian are most important. Horses with foot diseases should have farrier attention every 4 weeks.

Sometimes foot disease is unavoidable. Farriers are foot care specialists. A good working relationship between a competent farrier and veterinarian will assure that proper treatment is administered. The common goal of all is a sound, comfortable horse.

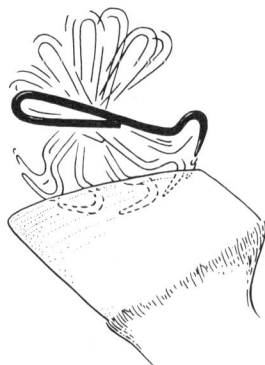

FOOT CARE MANNERS

Your horse's early training should include lessons in standing still for the shoeing process. Your trainer may use ropes and hobbles to teach this. It is best done as a part of the training process in a soft round pen as a part of the horse's ground training before riding or driving.

Foals can usually be restrained for trimming with a couple of assistants in a stall without hobbles. In fact, it is dangerous to restrain foals with hobbles due to the ease with which their bones break at the physis growth plates. Horses which have been trained from birth to give their feet for inspection will be easy to work with and won't harm themselves or the farrier. Give special attention to the balance of foals' feet to assure that their limbs are given a chance to grow straight. The farrier may nail or glue corrective shoes with extensions onto a baby's crooked feet.

Horses that have not been trained to stand still for shoeing may need to be disciplined by the farrier. Usually all that is required is a slap against the side with a leather popper. A twitch or lip chain may be necessary for persistent horses. Some may require further training with ropes or hobbles, and you should expect to pay extra for this service. Your farrier may request that a trainer handle the additional training. There is a chance that the horse and/or the farrier may be injured during the process. Untrained horses are a liability to everyone.

You can ensure that your horse will behave for the farrier by being firm with it between shoeings. Pick out its feet each time you ride. During your routine hoof inspection, tap the foot to imitate the farrier working. Do not allow the horse to take its foot from you at will. Be sure to have your horse trimmed or shod regularly according to its needs. Teach the horse patience by leaving it tied for extended periods. Restraint is often necessary to produce submissiveness in horses.

TRIMMING AND SHOEING

It takes a great deal of mental and physical effort to become a skilled farrier. Experience based on sound training is necessary. Most horse owners prefer to hire a professional to do their farrier work. Occasionally, horseowners may not be able to obtain a farrier and may chose to do routine hoof maintenance themselves. This requires special tools and training and a certain amount of physical strength.

Foot balance involves trimming and shoeing the hoof. Balance as it applies to horseshoeing may be defined as equal weight distribution around the center of gravity of the horse's limb. Foot balance is three-dimensional. It is divided into lateral/medial balance, hoof form balance, and hoof angle or toe/heel balance.

Balance is important when the horse is standing and when it is moving. There are two types of balance: *geometric balance* refers to the horse's conformation or stance when it is standing; *functional balance* refers to the balance during movement or gait. Geometric balance is the prime consideration that provides for the needs of most horses. Functional balance deals with speed horse shoeing and is often complicated.

Dressing the hoof, or forming with the rasp its lower two-thirds to be a continuation of the upper third, causes the distorted hoof to take the shape of the coffin bone.

Fitting the shoe involves placing it as close to the center of gravity of the limb as is practical. Perfect balance is rarely achieved but the closer we get to it, the better chance we have of maximizing performance and sustaining soundness in the horse.

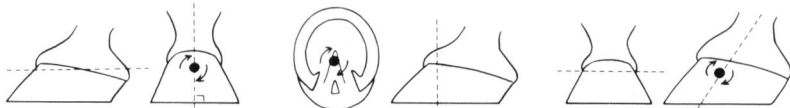

Balance is viewed from three perspectives.

SHOE SELECTION

Shoes come in many different sizes and styles. The heels of the shoe should cover the buttresses and give support at the heel of the foot. The style of the shoe may change according to the use of the horse and the season of the year.

Shoes are either handmade or machine-made. Most farriers use machine-made shoes due to the time involved in making handmade shoes. Using handmade shoes when machine-made ones are readily available is an expensive option. Shoes for special foot problems may need to be handmade if machine-made shoes are unavailable to create the ideal weight and effect for a particular foot.

Most machine-made shoes can be fit cold. Shoes with clips or rocker toes are usually fit hot to allow uniform seating of the shoe against the hoof. In addition, hot seating has been shown to have a beneficial effect on excessively moist and weak hoofs. Some horses may object to the smell of hot fitting, but it does not hurt them.

Shoe styles are named for the configuration of the stock section used to make the shoe. A plain flat shoe with fullering or creasing is used on most trail horses. Concave fullered shoes are popular for horses ridden on turf and in dirt arenas. Shoes with calks are traditional for mountain riding and packing. Polo plates and barrel racing shoes with high inner rims and high outer rims respectively are used on competition horses. Half-rounds are often used on young horses. Shoes can be tapped and removable calks, called studs, can be inserted.

Light weight shoes made from aluminum or titanium are popular for jumping horses. Racing plates made from aluminum are used on race horses. Wide webbed shoes are used on the hind feet of reining horses. Weighted shoes made from heavier stock are used to enhance the action of gaited show horses.

Farriers often use clips to stabilize shoes on weak hoofs. Rocker-toes are used to extend wear and ease the breakover on front hoofs. Square toes are used on hind hoofs to reduce the risk of injury from overreaching.

Bar shoes of various types are used as therapeutic shoes to treat various diseases of the feet. They apply or relieve pressure on various parts of the foot. Pads may be used in conjunction with shoes to protect sensitive areas of the hoof.

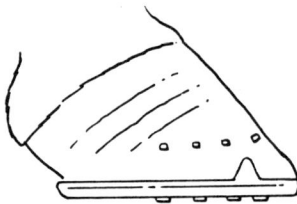

Side clip fit, side view

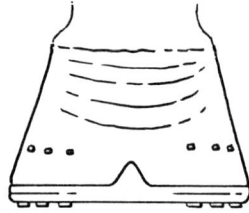

Toe clip fit, front view

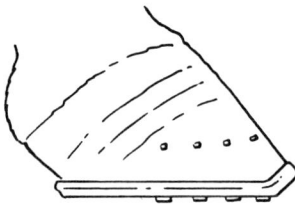

Rocker toe fit, side view

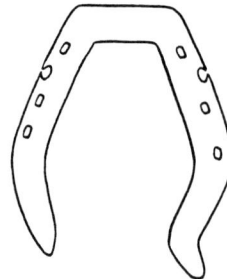

Stamped square toe with trailer & side clips

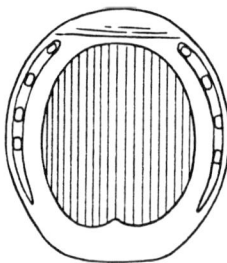

Egg bar shoe with pad

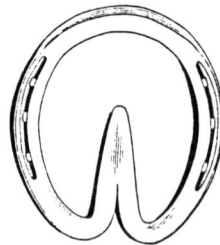

Heart bar shoe

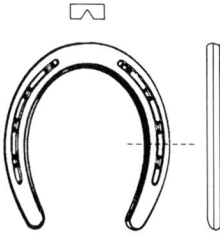

Flat-fullered plain

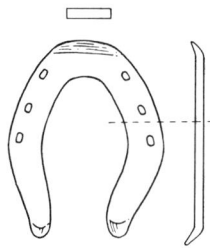

*Flat-stamped
reining plate*

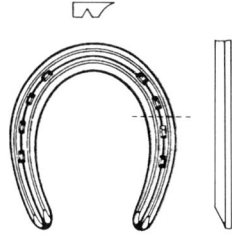

Concave-fullered rim

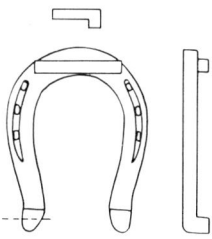

*Toe and heel calk
(mule shoe)*

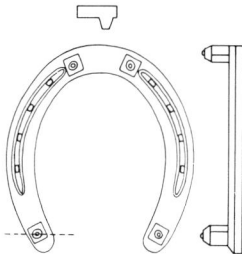

*Screw-in calks
or studs*

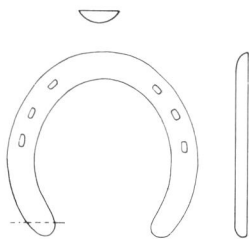

Half-round

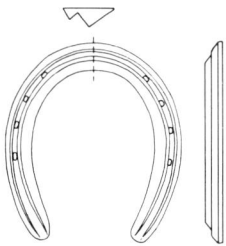

Polo plate

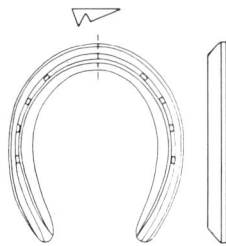

Barrel racing

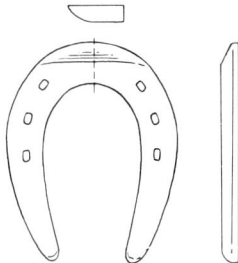

*Stamped toe weight with
rolled toe*

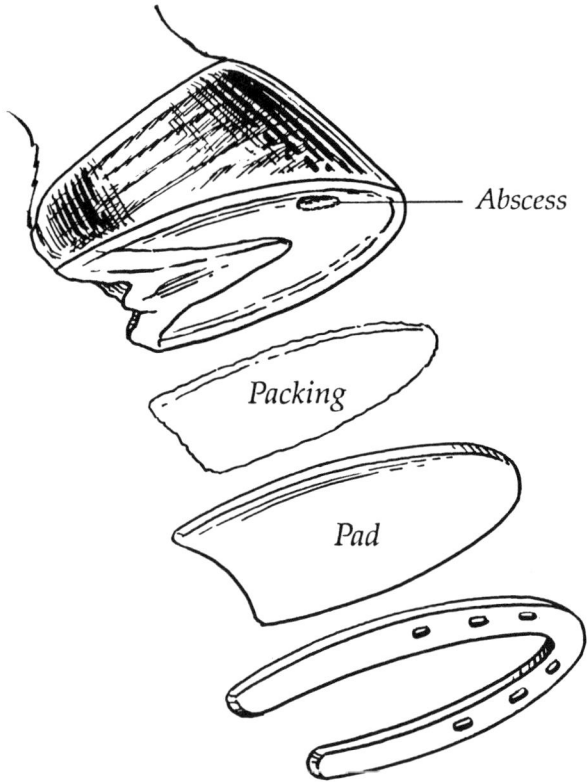

Pad application for a drained abscess.

FIRST AID

Horses (and horse persons) may be accidently injured in the course of daily activities. Knowing what to do in an emergency is essential. It is wise to be prepared before an accident or disease occurs. Keep an emergency kit containing medicines and tools on hand. The kit should include some horseshoeing tools such as: pull-offs/nail cutters, hoof knife, rasp, clinch cutter, driving hammer, and clinchers.

Have your horses vaccinated annually for tetanus and other diseases endemic to your area. Keep antiseptic preparations such as Furacin (nitrofurazone), Kopertox (copper sulfate), and poultices such as Ichthammol (20% back salve) and Epsom Salts (magnesium sulfate) readily available to assist veterinary medical treatment of foot ailments.

Bandaging material including gauze, Elastikon tape or Vetrap is useful for making foot bandages. You can use duct tape to protect a hoof when a shoe is thrown. Rolled cotton (cotton wool) is very useful in cleaning thrushy areas on the point of a hoof pick or to hold medication against the hoof under a bandage. Your veterinarian can advise you on what is needed for your individual situation.

Call your veterinarian immediately if your horse appears sick or has obvious pain. Advance preparation and first aid knowledge that can be applied before professional help arrives could save your horse's life.

Foot diseases may cause severe lameness and can be made worse by owner neglect. They sometimes occur even under optimum conditions. There are a few foot ailments that merit special attention due to their prevalence and severity. The least severe is thrush—the most severe is laminitis.

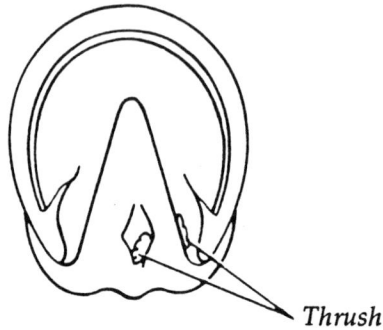

Thrush

The location of thrush in the foot.

THRUSH

Thrush is a destruction of the frog by the anaerobic bacteria, *Fusiforum necrophorum*. The infection is usually black and strong-smelling. It is located in the frog, most commonly in the commissure or sulcus. If the thrush infection is severe enough, it may penetrate the sensitive structures of the hoof and form an abscess.

Thrush in horses is often compared to athlete's foot in humans. Established infections may be difficult to dry up. Thrush usually stems from unclean, dirty conditions combined with long, untrimmed hoofs. Both conditions result from owner neglect. The dirty conditions provide an ideal environment for the anaerobic bacteria to grow. Cleaning out the foot once a day and exposing it to air as well as removing the infected areas will stop thrush. You can apply an antiseptic drying agent to help destroy any remaining bacteria. If you frequently clean out the horse's feet, have them trimmed or shod at least every six to eight weeks, and keep the horse in a well-drained lot, thrush is rarely a problem.

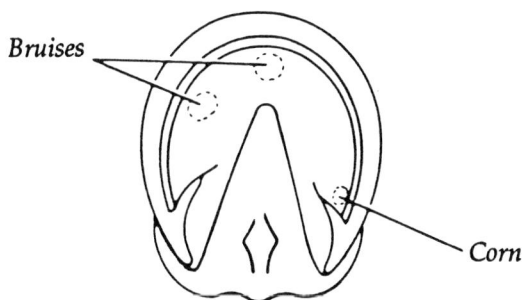

The location of sole bruises and a corn in the foot.

SOLE BRUISES

Sole bruises are caused by concussion to the sole. Sole bruises in the horse are similar to nail or bone bruises in humans. Injury can be caused by rocks, gravel, or other hard objects. An unlevel horseshoe may also cause sole bruises. A good preventative measure is to shoe horses that are to be ridden on gravel, rocks, or other hard surfaces. Once the sole is bruised, the horse should be shod if it is not already. Pads can also help protect the sole and relieve pain caused by the bruises. If the bruise is caused by the shoe, the offending shoe must be removed and a wide-webbed shoe that has been seated out on its inner foot surface should be applied.

Corns are specific types of sole bruises in the heel area of the foot. They are caused by leaving a short-heeled shoe on too long. Corns can usually be prevented by resetting the horse on schedule every six to eight weeks. Most corns can be improved by removing the shoe, trimming the hoof away from the bruised area, and applying a bar shoe to protect and transfer the weight bearing off the bruised area on to the frog. If a bruise is severe enough, it can develop into an abscess. Be aware of the situations that might lead to these conditions, and you will be able to prevent most sole bruising.

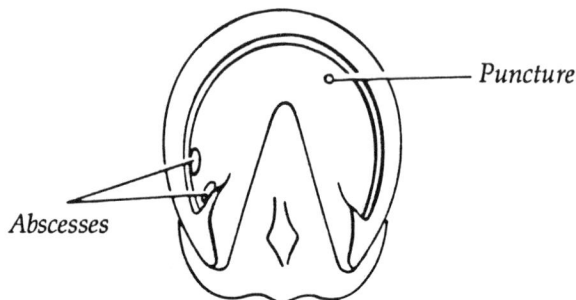

The location of abscesses in the foot.

ABSCESS

An abscess can cause intense pain and severe lameness. Prompt treatment by a competent farrier and veterinarian is critical.

An abscess is a pus pocket or an infection of the sensitive structures of the foot. It most commonly occurs in the sole or white line area of the hoof. An abscess is analogous to a boil or festered wound in humans. It may result from puncture wounds, thrush, sole bruises or laminitis. However, any openings in the sole or white line, even those caused by the natural expanison of the hoof, may allow bacteria to enter the sensitive structures and form an abscess.

An abscess follows the path of least resistance until it breaks out and drains, sometimes at the coronary band. To heal, it must be opened to allow drainage and drying. Soak the foot in Epsom salts to help promote drainage. Apply a germicide to the infected area to kill the remaining bacteria and dry the wound. Then pack the area with a poultice to encourage drainage. The farrier can then shoe the foot with a full pad under the shoe to protect the infected area or can construct a shoe with a removable plate so you can change packings and dressings. The shoe should be reset every four to six weeks.

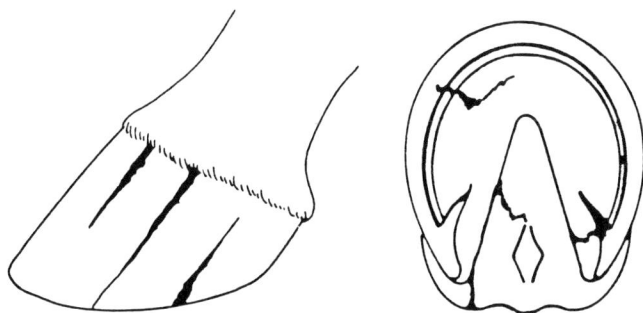

The location of sand cracks in the foot.

SAND CRACK

A sand crack (often called a toe or quarter crack, depending upon its location) is a vertical crack in the hoof wall. A crack can extend part way down the wall from the coronary band, part way up from the ground surface, or extend the full length of the wall. A hoof crack may be superficial and insignificant or deep and serious, causing intense pain. Toe cracks pinch when the foot bears weight. Quarter cracks hurt most when the foot is raised. Hoof cracks may result from uneven weight-bearing, irregular hoof growth, wire cuts, excessive hoof length, or dry conditions.

The sides of a crack will not heal and join together. They must be immobilized until the crack grows out like a torn fingernail. There are several methods available to treat sand cracks, including metal plates held in place by screws, bar shoes, shoe clips, metal hose clamps, lacing, and modern plastics. Great skill is needed to determine and apply the best method or combination of methods to repair a deep crack until it grows out. Shoes should be reset every four to six weeks.

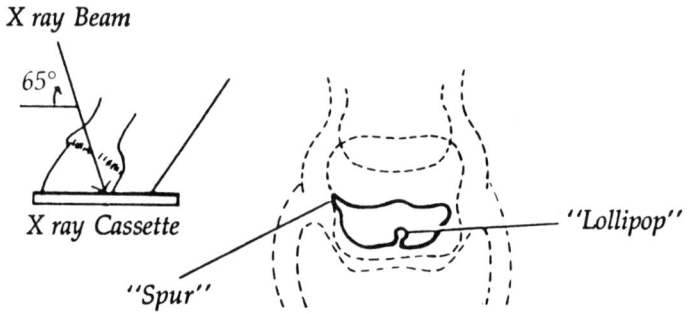

X ray Beam

65°

X ray Cassette

"Spur"

"Lollipop"

Lesions on the navicular bone that may be seen in a radiograph.

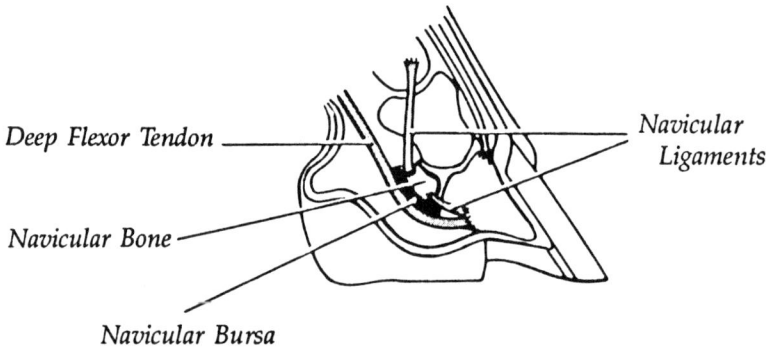

Deep Flexor Tendon

Navicular Bone

Navicular Bursa

Navicular Ligaments

The position of the navicular bone and its ligaments, bursa, and the deep flexor tendon.

NAVICULAR DISEASE

Navicular disease is the name given to pain in the area of the navicular bone. It may involve inflammation of the navicular bursa, ligament sprain, cartilage or tendon destruction, and bone changes. Pain may be mild or severe. Navicular disease in horses is similar to human athletic injuries due to over-exertion while being under-conditioned, which then develop into a progressive arthritis.

The navicular bone acts as a fulcrum point to redirect the pull of the deep flexor tendon against the coffin bone as the horse moves forward. The navicular bursa is a fluid-filled sack that lubricates the tendon surface of the navicular bone.

The navicular bone is held in place by two ligaments situated above and below the bone. Blood supply and nourishment come to the navicular bone through these ligaments. If these ligaments are injured from concussion (due to an excessively steep pastern) or compression (due to an excessively sloping pastern), lameness may occur and the blood supply to the navicular bone and its cartilage may be disrupted. Radiographs (X rays) may reveal "spurs" on the side(s) of the navicular bone or "lollipop" lesions on its base after the damage has occurred.

The signs of navicular disease include pointing the toe of the afflicted foot with the heel off the ground. Changes take place in the form of the hoof and it becomes contracted at the heel. The horse takes shorter steps when both front feet are affected. The horse will often warm

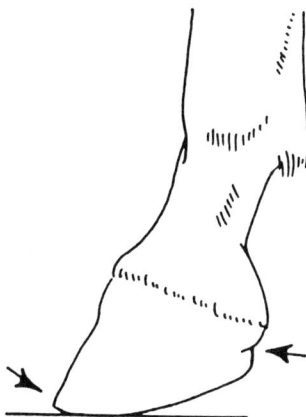

Signs of navicular disease.

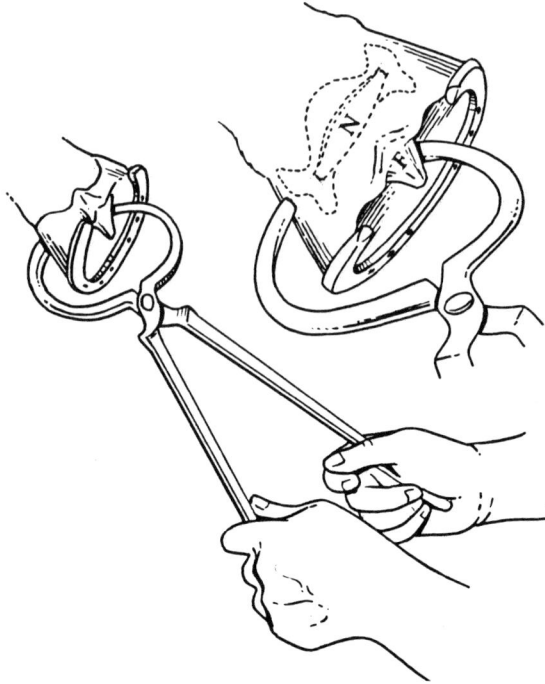

Hoof testers are used to diagnose navicular disease.

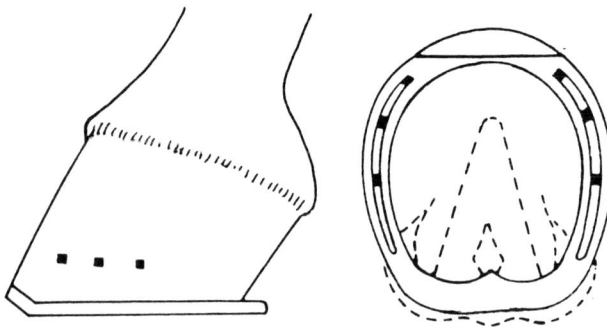

A bar shoe fit long with a rocker-toe is used to treat navicular disease.

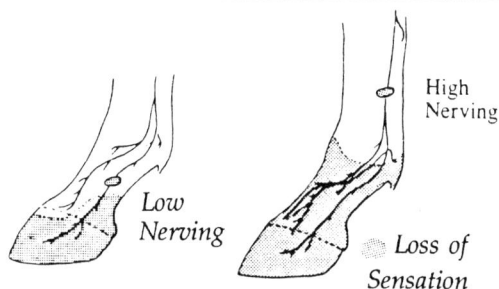

High
Nerving

*The effect of low
and high nerving.*

Low
Nerving

Loss of
Sensation

out of the lameness and will be worse after a period of rest.

The skilled use of hoof testers is the best method to diagnose navicular disease. The horse's response to pressure in specific areas of the hoof overlying the navicular bone is compared to that of a sound foot on the same horse. Nerve blocks and radiographs can be used to confirm the hoof testers' diagnosis.

The treatment for navicular disease is usually a bar shoe with heel support (length) and a rocker toe. The hoof is trimmed short in the toe. The object is to prevent strain on the deep flexor tendon and relieve pressure on the heel area to improve blood circulation. The shoes must be reset every four to six weeks in order to maintain the most beneficial hoof angle.

Occasionally, difficult cases may be most humanely handled by having the veterinarian do a low nerving operation. This is a treatment of last resort. Be aware that a nerved horse has no feeling in the back part of the foot and may unintentionally injure itself or the rider. Complications may develop. High nerving makes the horse even more dangerous and should be avoided.

Most horses which get navicular disease are predisposed to it by heredity or environmental conditions. The conformation of a horse's leg and foot affect susceptibility to navicular disease. Horses with small feet for their body size are especially susceptible. Lack of conditioning for the work performed is also a contributing cause. Navicular disease has become a common disease of stabled horses which are used occasionally for strenuous athletic activity.

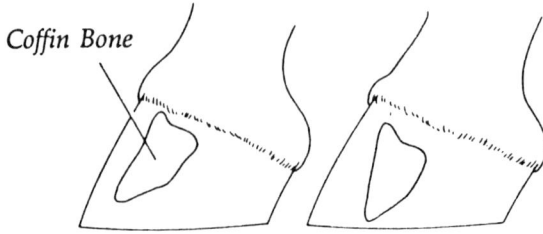

Coffin Bone

Death of the sensitive lamina allows the coffin bone to rotate or sink (founder) depending on the severity of the disease.

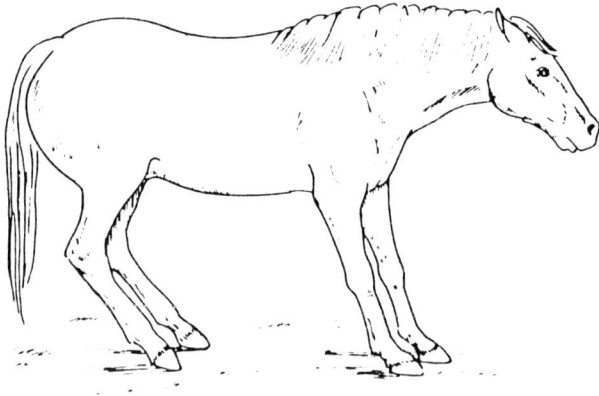

Characteristic laminitic stance.

LAMINITIS OR FOUNDER

Laminitis is the inflammation of the sensitive lamina of the hoof. It can be compared to a severe blood blister under a human fingernail. There are two types: *acute* and *chronic*.

Acute laminitis is a medical emergency and life-threatening situation. The sensitive lamina extending from the bone at the toe will die very shortly after onset. The horny lamina of the wall then separates from the sensitive lamina at the coffin bone which allows the coffin bone to rotate or sink (founder). Radiographs (X rays) reveal the movement of the bone. If it is not stabilized, it may penetrate the bottom of the sole. The subsequent infection and pain may cause the horse's death.

Acute laminitis is caused by some type of stress to the horse's system. Possibilities include excessive grain intake or cold water intake, changes in feeds or feeding routine, excessive concussion or fatigue, infections or poisons, and drug abuse or allergies.

Signs of acute laminitis include heat in the foot with a stronger than normal digital pulse and a characteristic stance. The horse stands with its front feet extended forward and rocks back onto the hind feet, drawing them under its body for support.

Treatment is very difficult and often disappointing. The animal's system must be medically stabilized so it can repair itself. The coffin bone must be stabilized to prevent its further rotating or sinking and eventually puncturing the sole. The foot infection (abscesses) must be drained and the foot kept clean and hoof kept pliable. Part of the hoof wall may need to be removed initially to allow effective treatment. The purpose of these procedures is to improve the circulation in the foot to aid in the repair of damage caused by the disease. It may take as much as a year of daily treatments before a horse fully recovers. Many never totally recover and some die even with the best of care. Treatments must involve both the farrier and the veterinarian.

The research of Dr. Chris Pollitt of Australia has shown that some form of frog support is necessary to re-establish blood circulation at the toe of a foundered horse.

The experience of Burney Chapman of Texas and Dr. Robert Eustace of England, indicates that properly applied frog support (heart bar shoes) provides the greatest chance for successful outcome.

Heart bar shoes apply support to the forward third of the frog to help stabilize the coffin bone. They should be reset every three to four weeks to maintain the most beneficial support pressure and proper alignment of the bones. Radiographs are used to determine the exact fitting of the shoe. Early in treatment, drugs may be used to deaden pain and improve the circulation in the foot. Forced exercise may be recommended in later states of treatment. Daily nursing care and bandages may be necessary for months in many cases.

Chronic laminitis produces a lingering lameness that limits a horse's usefulness. Avoid purchasing horses which have chronic laminitis. Check for irregular rings in the hoof wall that are wider at the heel than at the toe, a wide white line at the toe, and a flat sole on the bottom of the hoof. Animals with chronic laminitis may develop the acute form of the disease when subjected to stressful conditions.

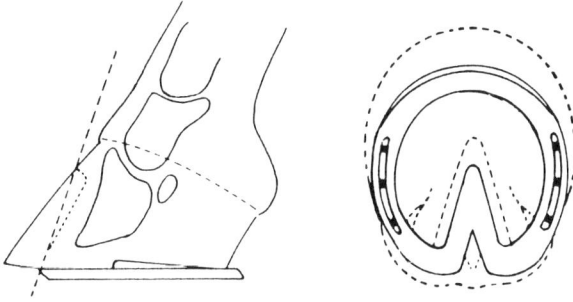

A heart bar shoe is fit with pressure on the forward third of the frog to help
stabilize the coffin bone. The deformed hoof is rasped away.
Abscesses must be opened and drained at the toe.

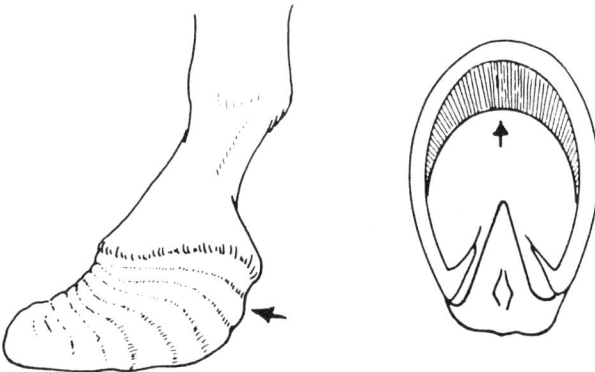

Signs that indicate chronic laminitis.

FARRIER SELECTION

Selecting a farrier is one of the most important decisions you will make regarding horse care. You may be fortunate to live in an area where there are several good farriers to choose from. In some areas, there may be only one person available. Lack of choice has caused some horse owners to attend a farrier school and learn to do this work. However, most people will switch to a competent, dependable farrier as soon as one is available.

As a horse owner, you must learn how to recognize good work. Differences in gait caused by shoeing changes may be very subtle. It is best to see the farrier's work on another person's horse and to get a recommendation from a respected horse person before selecting a farrier for your valuable animals.

Basing your farrier selection only on the farrier school's certificate can be risky. Most of these are simply certificates of completion which certify that the person attended the school. Schools vary tremendously in their programs, and they are only the beginning for any farrier. Additional experience as well as regular attendance at clinics is essential to keep skills and knowledge current. People vary in their ability to absorb new information and to develop the eye-hand coordination necessary to become an accomplished farrier. Don't hesitate to ask your prospective farrier about his or her experience and training, especially as it relates to your animals.

There are no skill tests required by government agencies in the United States to become a farrier. The selection of the farrier is up to you. Certification by a regional farrier organization is helpful and indicates that the farrier is willing to subject his or her skill to peer review. As with many services, a solid recommendation from a satisfied client is of supreme importance.

The more you know about the process of horseshoeing and the options available, the better chance you have of giving your horse optimum hoof care. Work closely with your farrier and your veterinarian; ask questions and follow through on their suggestions and recommendations. If you'd like to learn more, the textbook *The Principles of Horseshoeing II* is a good place to start.

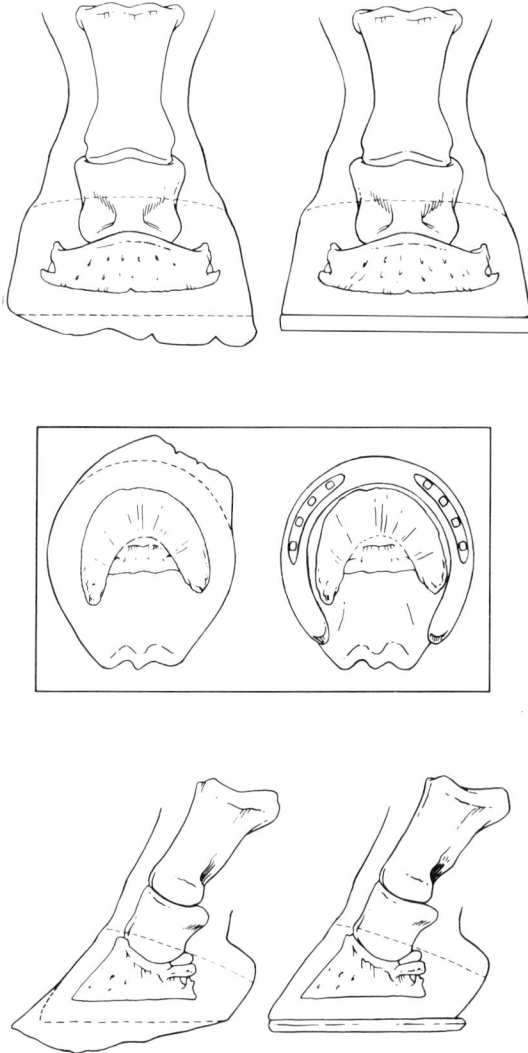

Before and after balance, showing position of the coffin bone.

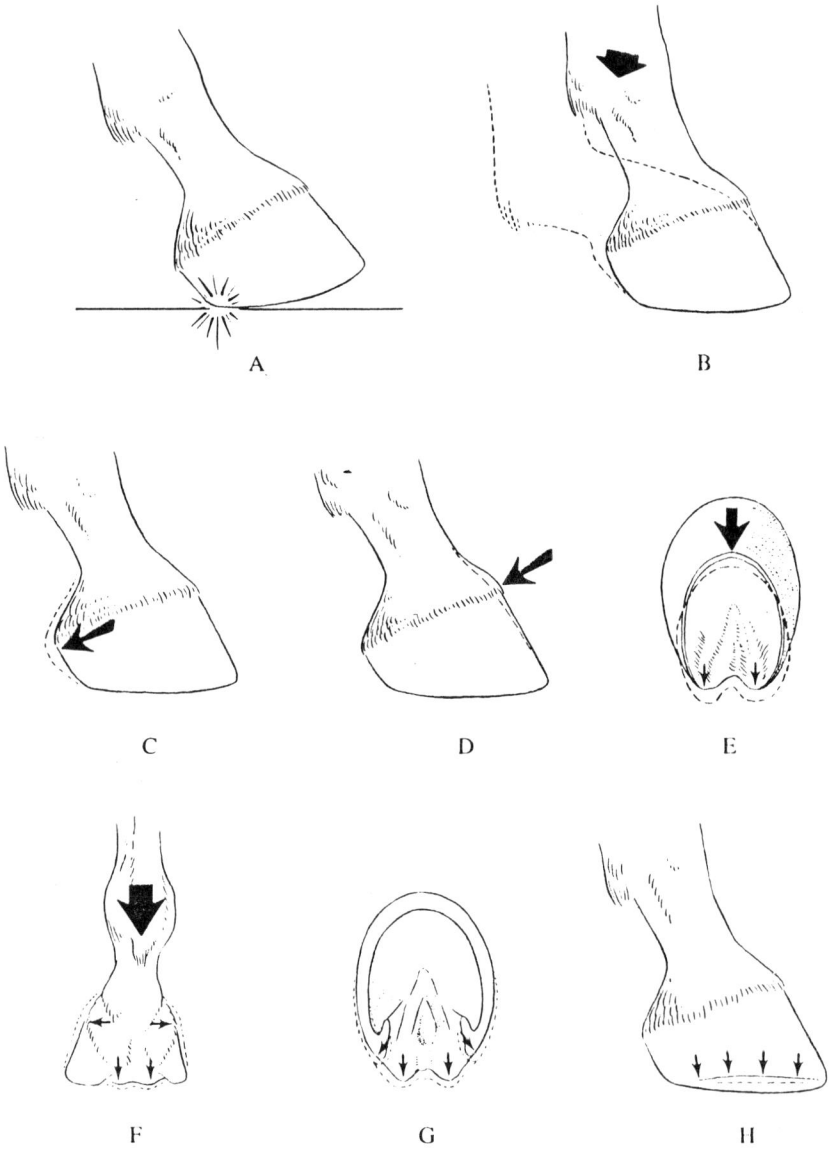

Hoof movement during weight-bearing

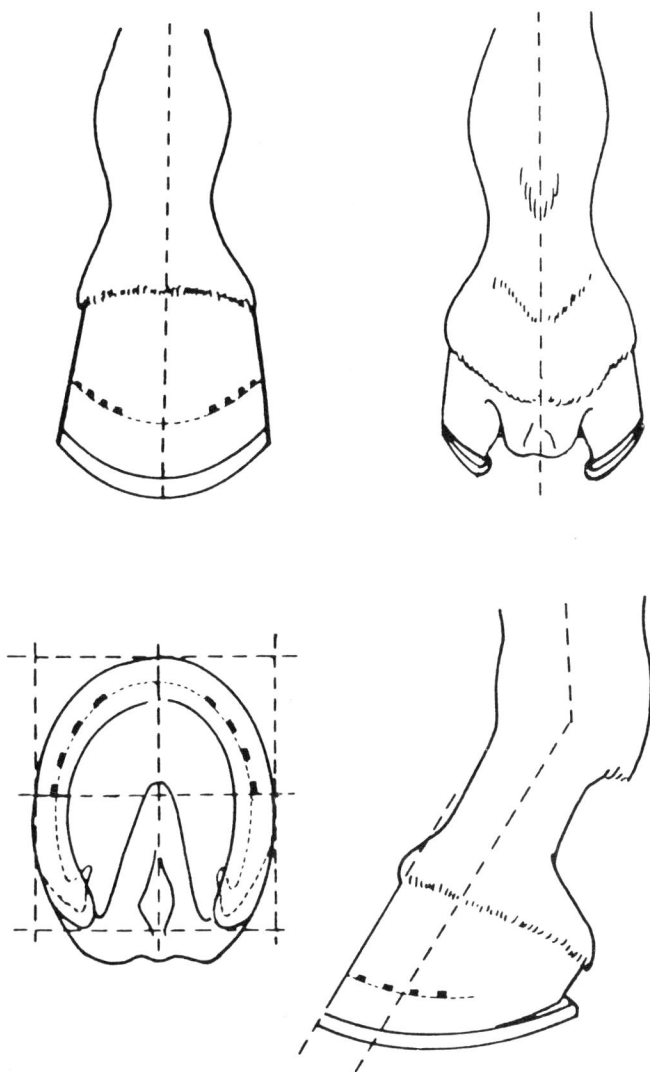

A well-balanced foot.

Toe

Web

Outer Rim

Toe Nail Hole
(1st Nail Hole)

Inner Rim

Quarter Nail
Holes (2nd
& 3rd Nail
Holes)

Crease
or
Fullering

Branch

Heel Nail
Hole (Last
Nail Hole)

Concaving

Area of
Expansion

Heels

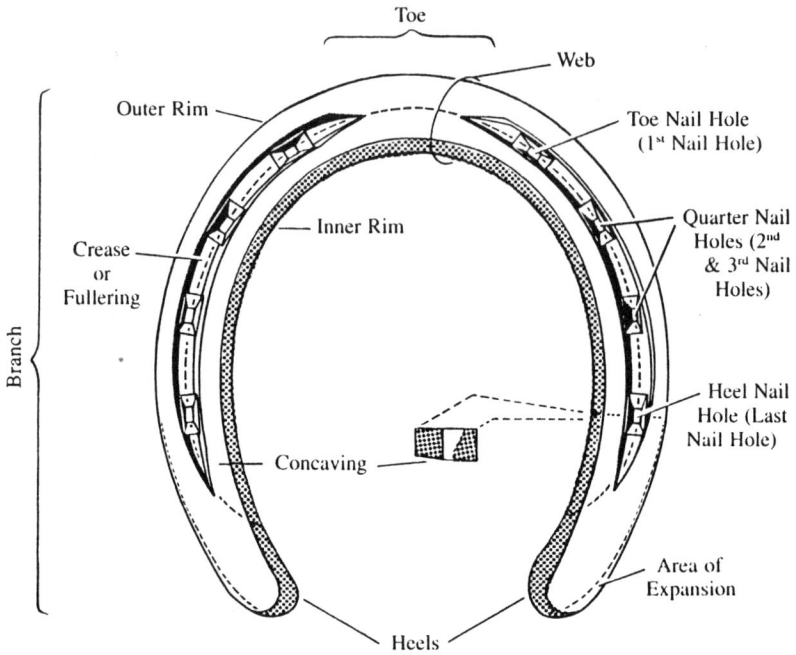

Projects from Shoe

Buried in Shoe

Head

Neck

Bevel of
Head

Buried in Hoof Wall

Inner Face

Blade
or
Shank

Clinch

Outer Face

Wrung Off

Bevel of
Point

Point

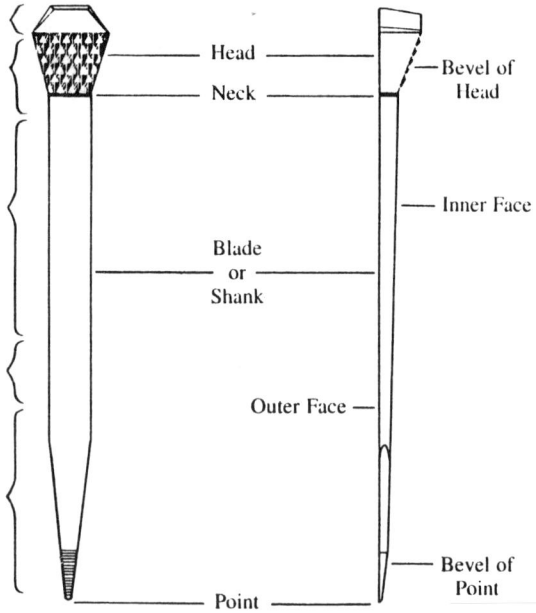

**The Parts of the
Shoe and Nail**